30-DAY MACRO DIET MEAL PLAN

Delicious, Nutritious, and Balanced Meals to Help You Reach Your Goals

Dr Lily Morgan

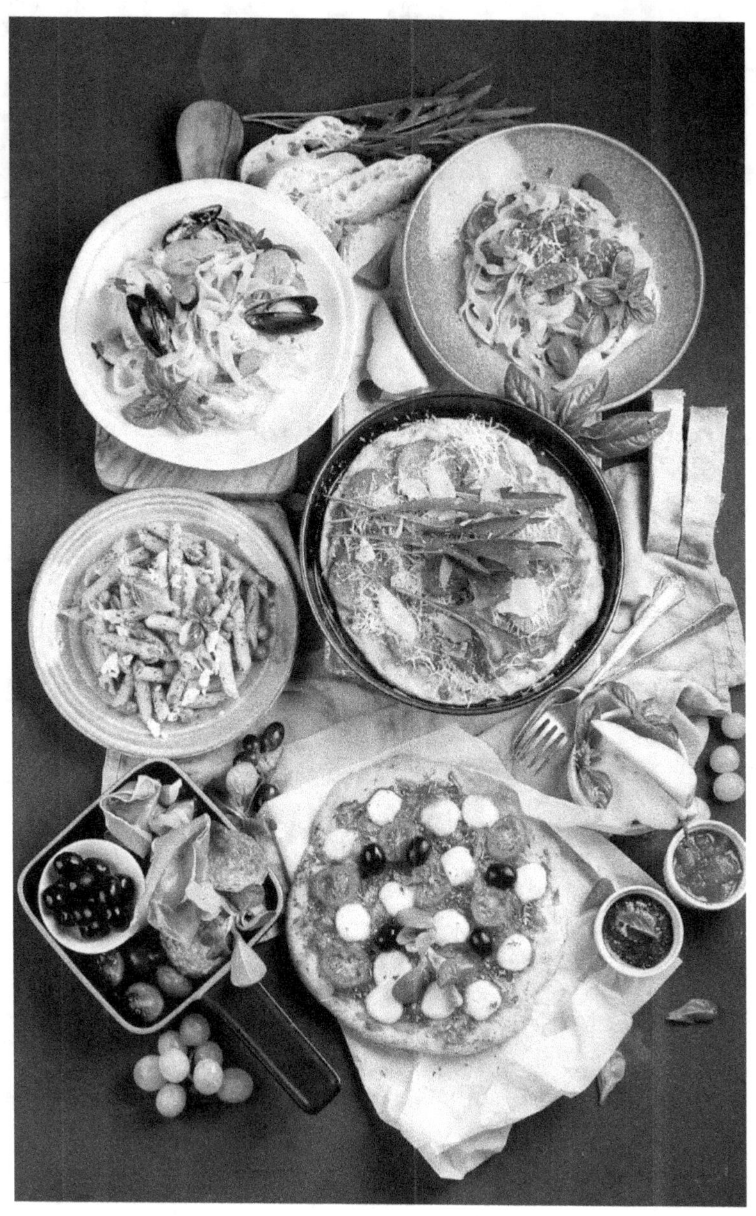

TABLE OF CONTENTS

Chapter 3: Lunch Recipes..41

Chapter 4: Dinner Recipes 55

Chapter 5: Snacks and Appetizers 72

INTRODUCTION

The journey to better health and wellness often begins with understanding the importance of proper nutrition and its impact on our bodies. In this introductory chapter, we will delve into the world of healthful eating and explore the concept of the macro diet.

The Quest for Optimal Health

From ancient civilizations to modern times, the quest for optimal health has been a driving force behind human existence. We have always sought ways to nourish our bodies, enhance our well-being, and extend our lifespans. Throughout history, various dietary practices have emerged, each promising unique benefits and solutions to our health concerns.

As we navigate the complexities of the modern world, with its abundance of processed foods and sedentary lifestyles, the need for a balanced and sustainable approach to eating has never been greater. Enter the macro diet, a nutritional philosophy that emphasizes the significance of macronutrients in our daily meals.

Understanding the Macro Diet

At its core, the macro diet centers around the three essential macronutrients: carbohydrates, proteins, and fats. These nutrients form the foundation of our diet and provide us with the energy needed to fuel our activities, support bodily functions, and maintain overall well-being.

Carbohydrates: Often regarded as the body's primary source of energy, carbohydrates come in various forms, from simple sugars found in fruits to complex carbohydrates in whole grains. The macro diet encourages the consumption of wholesome, unprocessed carbohydrates to sustain steady energy levels and prevent spikes in blood sugar.

Proteins: Vital for growth, repair, and maintenance of tissues, proteins are the building blocks of life. They play a crucial role in muscle development, immune function, and enzyme production. In the macro diet, adequate protein intake is promoted to support the body's repair and rejuvenation processes.

Fats: Contrary to popular belief, fats are not the enemy. In fact, they are essential for the absorption of certain vitamins, hormone production, and brain function. The macro diet emphasizes the consumption of healthy fats, such as those found in avocados, nuts, and olive oil, while limiting trans fats and saturated fats.

Benefits of the Macro Diet

The macro diet offers a plethora of potential benefits for those who adopt it as a lifestyle choice. Some of the notable advantages include:

- **Weight Management**: By focusing on macronutrient balance and portion control, the macro diet can be an effective tool for weight management and body composition improvement.
- **Sustainable Approach:** Unlike restrictive diets that often lead to temporary results, the macro diet promotes a sustainable approach to eating. It allows

for flexibility and can be customized to suit individual preferences and dietary restrictions.

- **Enhanced Energy Levels**: With a balanced intake of macronutrients, individuals on the macro diet often report improved energy levels throughout the day, reducing the need for frequent snacking.
- **Blood Sugar Regulation**: By choosing nutrient-dense, low-glycemic foods, the macro diet can help stabilize blood sugar levels, reducing the risk of diabetes and promoting better insulin sensitivity.
- **Muscle Preservation:** Adequate protein intake in the macro diet helps preserve lean muscle mass, particularly important for those engaged in physical activities and exercise routines.
- **Increased Nutrient Intake**: Emphasizing whole, nutrient-rich foods ensures that followers of the macro diet receive a wide array of vitamins, minerals, and antioxidants that support overall health.

How to Follow the 30-Day Macro Diet Meal Plan

Embarking on the 30-day macro diet meal plan requires dedication, planning, and a commitment to making healthier choices. Here are some key steps to follow the plan successfully:

- **Set Clear Goals:** Define your objectives for adopting the macro diet. Whether it's weight loss, improved energy, or better overall health, having specific goals will keep you motivated throughout the journey.
- **Calculate Your Macros**: Consult with a nutritionist or use online tools to determine your ideal macronutrient ratios based on factors like age, gender, weight, activity level, and goals.
- **Meal Preparation:** Planning and preparing meals in advance will help you stay on track and avoid unhealthy food choices when hunger strikes.
- **Stay Hydrated:** Water plays a crucial role in digestion, nutrient absorption, and overall health.

Aim to drink enough water throughout the day to stay adequately hydrated.

- **Practice Portion Control**: While the macro diet is flexible, portion control is essential to ensure you're meeting your macro targets and not overindulging in any specific nutrient.

- **Be Mindful of Snacks:** Snacking can add up quickly in terms of calorie and macro intake. Choose nutrient-dense snacks and be mindful of their contribution to your daily goals.

- **Track Progress:** Keeping a food journal or using a mobile app can help you track your meals, macros, and progress throughout the 30-day journey.

Chapter 1: 30 Day Meal Plan

Week 1: Daily Meal

Day 1:

Breakfast: Protein-Packed Omelette with Veggies

Lunch: Grilled Chicken Salad with Balsamic Vinaigrette

Dinner: Baked Salmon with Asparagus and Lemon

Snack: Veggie Sticks with Hummus

Dessert: Mixed Berry Parfait with Greek Yogurt

Day 2:

Breakfast: Greek Yogurt Parfait with Berries and Granola

Lunch: Black Bean and Quinoa Salad

Dinner: Lemon Herb Grilled Chicken with Roasted
Vegetables

Snack: Greek Yogurt with Cucumber and Dill Dip

Dessert: Chocolate Protein Balls with Almond Butter

Day 3:

Breakfast: Quinoa Breakfast Bowl with Almonds and
Honey

Lunch: Turkey and Avocado Wrap

Dinner: Spaghetti Squash with Marinara and Turkey Meatballs

Snack: Sliced Apple with Almond Butter

Dessert: Frozen Banana Popsicles with Dark Chocolate Drizzle

Day 4:

Breakfast: Avocado Toast with Poached Eggs

Lunch: Mediterranean Chickpea Salad

Dinner: Zucchini Noodles with Pesto and Cherry Tomatoes

Snack: Rice Cakes with Avocado and Sprouts

Dessert: Baked Apples with Cinnamon and Greek Yogurt

Day 5:

Breakfast: Veggie and Cheese Frittata

Lunch: Shrimp and Veggie Stir-Fry

Dinner: Beef Stir-Fry with Broccoli and Snow Peas

Snack: Edamame with Sea Salt

Dessert: Chia Seed Chocolate Pudding

Day 6:

Breakfast: Chia Seed Pudding with Mixed Fruits

Lunch: Tofu Lettuce Wraps with Peanut Sauce

Dinner: Cauliflower Rice Stir-Fry with Tofu and Cashews

Snack: Guacamole and Salsa with Baked Tortilla Chips

Dessert: Coconut and Date Energy Bites

Day 7:

Breakfast: Banana Nut Smoothie Bowl

Lunch: Lentil and Vegetable Soup

Dinner: Stuffed Bell Peppers with Quinoa and Black Beans

Snack: Cottage Cheese and Pineapple Chunks

Dessert: Peanut Butter and Banana Frozen Bites

Week 2: Daily Meal

Day 8:

Breakfast: Cottage Cheese Pancakes with Blueberry Compote

Lunch: Turkey and Sweet Potato Chili

Dinner: Baked Cod with Steamed Green Beans

Snack: Mixed Nuts and Seeds Trail Mix

Dessert: Berry Chia Seed Jam on Whole Grain Toast

Day 9:

Breakfast: Spinach and Mushroom Breakfast Burrito

Lunch: Falafel Bowl with Hummus and Tabouli

Dinner: Eggplant Parmesan with Mixed Greens Salad

Snack: Carrot and Zucchini Fritters

Dessert: Almond Flour Chocolate Chip Cookies

Day 10:

Breakfast: Almond Butter and Banana Sandwich on Whole Grain Bread

Lunch: Grilled Portobello Mushroom Burger

Dinner: Thai Green Curry with Tofu and Cauliflower Rice

Snack: Stuffed Mini Bell Peppers with Goat Cheese

Dessert: Greek Yogurt and Mixed Berries Sorbet

Day 11:

Breakfast: Protein-Packed Omelette with Veggies

Lunch: Grilled Chicken Salad with Balsamic Vinaigrette

Dinner: Baked Salmon with Asparagus and Lemon

Snack: Veggie Sticks with Hummus

Dessert: Mixed Berry Parfait with Greek Yogurt

Day 12:

Breakfast: Greek Yogurt Parfait with Berries and Granola

Lunch: Black Bean and Quinoa Salad

Dinner: Lemon Herb Grilled Chicken with Roasted
Vegetables

Snack: Greek Yogurt with Cucumber and Dill Dip

Dessert: Chocolate Protein Balls with Almond Butter

Day 13:

Breakfast: Quinoa Breakfast Bowl with Almonds and
Honey

Lunch: Turkey and Avocado Wrap

Dinner: Spaghetti Squash with Marinara and Turkey
Meatballs

Snack: Sliced Apple with Almond Butter

Dessert: Frozen Banana Popsicles with Dark Chocolate
Drizzle

Day 14:

Breakfast: Avocado Toast with Poached Eggs

Lunch: Mediterranean Chickpea Salad

Dinner: Zucchini Noodles with Pesto and Cherry Tomatoes

Snack: Rice Cakes with Avocado and Sprouts

Dessert: Baked Apples with Cinnamon and Greek Yogurt

Week 3: Daily Meal

Day 15:

Breakfast: Veggie and Cheese Frittata

Lunch: Shrimp and Veggie Stir-Fry

Dinner: Beef Stir-Fry with Broccoli and Snow Peas

Snack: Edamame with Sea Salt

Dessert: Chia Seed Chocolate Pudding

Day 16:

Breakfast: Chia Seed Pudding with Mixed Fruits

Lunch: Tofu Lettuce Wraps with Peanut Sauce

Dinner: Cauliflower Rice Stir-Fry with Tofu and Cashews

Snack: Guacamole and Salsa with Baked Tortilla Chips

Dessert: Coconut and Date Energy Bites

Day 17:

Breakfast: Banana Nut Smoothie Bowl

Lunch: Lentil and Vegetable Soup

Dinner: Stuffed Bell Peppers with Quinoa and Black Beans

Snack: Cottage Cheese and Pineapple Chunks

Dessert: Peanut Butter and Banana Frozen Bites

Day 18:

Breakfast: Cottage Cheese Pancakes with Blueberry
Compote

Lunch: Turkey and Sweet Potato Chili

Dinner: Baked Cod with Steamed Green Beans

Snack: Mixed Nuts and Seeds Trail Mix

Dessert: Berry Chia Seed Jam on Whole Grain Toast

Day 19:

Breakfast: Spinach and Mushroom Breakfast Burrito

Lunch: Falafel Bowl with Hummus and Tabouli

Dinner: Eggplant Parmesan with Mixed Greens Salad

Snack: Carrot and Zucchini Fritters

Dessert: Almond Flour Chocolate Chip Cookies

Day 20:

Breakfast: Almond Butter and Banana Sandwich on Whole
Grain Bread

Lunch: Grilled Portobello Mushroom Burger

Dinner: Thai Green Curry with Tofu and Cauliflower Rice

Snack: Stuffed Mini Bell Peppers with Goat Cheese

Dessert: Greek Yogurt and Mixed Berries Sorbet

Day 21:

Breakfast: Protein-Packed Omelette with Veggies

Lunch: Grilled Chicken Salad with Balsamic Vinaigrette

Dinner: Baked Salmon with Asparagus and Lemon

Snack: Veggie Sticks with Hummus

Dessert: Mixed Berry Parfait with Greek Yogurt

Week 4: Daily Meal

Day 22:

Breakfast: Greek Yogurt Parfait with Berries and Granola

Lunch: Black Bean and Quinoa Salad

Dinner: Lemon Herb Grilled Chicken with Roasted Vegetables

Snack: Greek Yogurt with Cucumber and Dill Dip

Dessert: Chocolate Protein Balls with Almond Butter

Day 23:

Breakfast: Quinoa Breakfast Bowl with Almonds and Honey

Lunch: Turkey and Avocado Wrap

Dinner: Spaghetti Squash with Marinara and Turkey Meatballs

Snack: Sliced Apple with Almond Butter

Dessert: Frozen Banana Popsicles with Dark Chocolate Drizzle

Day 24:

Breakfast: Avocado Toast with Poached Eggs

Lunch: Mediterranean Chickpea Salad

Dinner: Zucchini Noodles with Pesto and Cherry Tomatoes

Snack: Rice Cakes with Avocado and Sprouts

Dessert: Baked Apples with Cinnamon and Greek Yogurt

Day 25:

Breakfast: Veggie and Cheese Frittata

Lunch: Shrimp and Veggie Stir-Fry

Dinner: Beef Stir-Fry with Broccoli and Snow Peas

Snack: Edamame with Sea Salt

Dessert: Chia Seed Chocolate Pudding

Day 26:

Breakfast: Chia Seed Pudding with Mixed Fruits

Lunch: Tofu Lettuce Wraps with Peanut Sauce

Dinner: Cauliflower Rice Stir-Fry with Tofu and Cashews

Snack: Guacamole and Salsa with Baked Tortilla Chips

Dessert: Coconut and Date Energy Bites

Day 27:

Breakfast: Banana Nut Smoothie Bowl

Lunch: Lentil and Vegetable Soup

Dinner: Stuffed Bell Peppers with Quinoa and Black Beans

Snack: Cottage Cheese and Pineapple Chunks

Dessert: Peanut Butter and Banana Frozen Bites

Day 28:

Breakfast: Cottage Cheese Pancakes with Blueberry Compote

Lunch: Turkey and Sweet Potato Chili

Dinner: Baked Cod with Steamed Green Beans

Snack: Mixed Nuts and Seeds Trail Mix

Dessert: Berry Chia Seed Jam on Whole Grain Toast

Day 29:

Breakfast: Spinach and Mushroom Breakfast Burrito

Lunch: Falafel Bowl with Hummus and Tabouli

Dinner: Eggplant Parmesan with Mixed Greens Salad

Snack: Carrot and Zucchini Fritters

Dessert: Almond Flour Chocolate Chip Cookies

Day 30:

Breakfast: Almond Butter and Banana Sandwich on Whole Grain Bread

Lunch: Grilled Portobello Mushroom Burger

Dinner: Thai Green Curry with Tofu and Cauliflower Rice

Snack: Stuffed Mini Bell Peppers with Goat Cheese

Dessert: Greek Yogurt and Mixed Berries Sorbet

Chapter 2: Breakfast Recipes

In this chapter, we will explore delicious and nutritious breakfast recipes to kickstart your day with energy and vitality. Each recipe is carefully crafted to provide a balanced mix of essential macronutrients while tantalizing your taste buds.

Protein-Packed Omelette with Veggies

Ingredients:

- 4 large eggs
- 1/4 cup diced bell peppers (red, green, or yellow)
- 1/4 cup diced onions
- 1/4 cup sliced mushrooms
- 1/4 cup chopped spinach
- 1/4 cup diced tomatoes
- 1/4 cup shredded cheddar cheese
- Salt and pepper to taste
- 1 tablespoon olive oil

Instructions:

1. In a medium-sized bowl, whisk the eggs until well beaten. Season with salt and pepper according to your taste.
2. Heat the olive oil in a non-stick skillet over medium heat.
3. Add the diced bell peppers and onions to the skillet and sauté until they become tender.
4. Stir in the sliced mushrooms and chopped spinach, cooking until the spinach wilts.
5. Pour the beaten eggs over the sautéed vegetables, ensuring an even distribution.
6. Sprinkle the diced tomatoes and shredded cheddar cheese over the omelette.
7. Cook the omelette for about 2-3 minutes or until the edges are set.
8. Carefully fold the omelette in half using a spatula and continue to cook for an additional minute until the cheese is melted.
9. Slide the omelette onto a plate and serve hot.

Greek Yogurt Parfait with Berries and Granola

Ingredients:

- 1 cup Greek yogurt
- 1/2 cup mixed berries (strawberries, blueberries, raspberries)
- 1/4 cup granola
- 1 tablespoon honey
- Fresh mint leaves for garnish (optional)

Instructions:

1. In a glass or a small bowl, layer the Greek yogurt, mixed berries, and granola.
2. Drizzle honey over the top of the parfait for added sweetness.
3. Garnish with fresh mint leaves, if desired.
4. Serve immediately and enjoy this delicious and nutritious breakfast treat!

Quinoa Breakfast Bowl with Almonds and Honey

Ingredients:

- 1 cup cooked quinoa
- 1/4 cup almond milk
- 1/4 cup sliced almonds
- 1 tablespoon honey
- 1/2 teaspoon ground cinnamon
- Fresh berries for topping

Instructions:

1. In a small saucepan, warm the almond milk over low heat.
2. Stir in the cooked quinoa, sliced almonds, honey, and ground cinnamon.
3. Cook the mixture for 2-3 minutes, stirring occasionally, until it reaches the desired consistency.
4. Transfer the quinoa breakfast bowl to a serving dish and top with fresh berries.
5. Drizzle a little extra honey on top for added sweetness if desired.

6. Enjoy this hearty and wholesome breakfast to start your day right.

Avocado Toast with Poached Eggs

Ingredients:

- 2 slices whole grain bread, toasted
- 1 ripe avocado, mashed
- 2 large eggs
- Salt and pepper to taste
- Fresh chives or cilantro for garnish (optional)

Instructions:

1. Poach the eggs: Fill a medium-sized saucepan with water and bring it to a simmer over medium heat.
2. Crack one egg into a small bowl. Create a gentle whirlpool in the simmering water using a spoon, and carefully slide the egg into the center of the whirlpool.
3. Poach the egg for about 3-4 minutes or until the white is set but the yolk is still runny. Remove the poached egg with a slotted spoon and set it aside on a plate.

4. Repeat the poaching process with the second egg.

5. Spread the mashed avocado evenly on the toasted bread slices.

6. Place one poached egg on each slice of avocado toast.

7. Season with salt and pepper to taste.

8. Garnish with fresh chives or cilantro if desired.

9. Serve immediately and enjoy this satisfying and nutritious breakfast.

Veggie and Cheese Frittata

Ingredients:

- 6 large eggs
- 1/4 cup milk
- 1/2 cup diced bell peppers (red, green, or yellow)
- 1/4 cup diced onions
- 1/4 cup sliced mushrooms
- 1/4 cup chopped spinach
- 1/4 cup diced tomatoes
- 1/2 cup shredded cheddar cheese
- Salt and pepper to taste
- 1 tablespoon olive oil

Instructions:

1. Preheat the oven to 350°F (175°C).

2. In a medium-sized bowl, whisk the eggs and milk until well combined. Season with salt and pepper according to your taste.

3. Heat the olive oil in an oven-safe skillet over medium heat.

4. Add the diced bell peppers and onions to the skillet and sauté until they become tender.

5. Stir in the sliced mushrooms and chopped spinach, cooking until the spinach wilts.

6. Pour the beaten egg mixture over the sautéed vegetables, ensuring an even distribution.

7. Sprinkle the diced tomatoes and shredded cheddar cheese over the frittata.

8. Transfer the skillet to the preheated oven and bake for 15-20 minutes or until the frittata is set and slightly golden on top.

9. Remove the skillet from the oven and let it cool slightly.

10. Cut the frittata into wedges and serve hot.

Chia Seed Pudding with Mixed Fruits

Ingredients:

- 1/4 cup chia seeds
- 1 cup almond milk
- 1 tablespoon honey or maple syrup
- 1/2 teaspoon vanilla extract
- Mixed fruits (such as berries, kiwi, and mango) for topping

Instructions:

1. In a medium-sized bowl, whisk together the chia seeds, almond milk, honey or maple syrup, and vanilla extract until well combined.
2. Cover the bowl and refrigerate the mixture for at least 2 hours or overnight to allow the chia seeds to expand and create a pudding-like texture.
3. Before serving, give the chia seed pudding a good stir.
4. Top the pudding with mixed fruits for a burst of flavor and color.
5. Serve this delightful and nutritious chia seed pudding for a refreshing breakfast.

Banana Nut Smoothie Bowl

Ingredients:

- 2 ripe bananas, peeled and frozen
- 1/2 cup almond milk
- 1/4 cup Greek yogurt
- 2 tablespoons almond butter
- 1 tablespoon honey
- 1/4 cup granola
- 1 tablespoon chopped nuts (such as almonds, walnuts, or pecans)
- Sliced bananas and berries for topping

Instructions:

1. In a blender, combine the frozen bananas, almond milk, Greek yogurt, almond butter, and honey.
2. Blend until smooth and creamy, adding more almond milk if needed to achieve the desired consistency.
3. Pour the banana nut smoothie into a bowl.
4. Top the smoothie with granola, chopped nuts, sliced bananas, and berries.

5. Drizzle a little extra honey on top for added sweetness if desired.

6. Enjoy this delicious and filling smoothie bowl for a nourishing breakfast.

Cottage Cheese Pancakes with Blueberry Compote

Ingredients:

- 1 cup cottage cheese
- 3 large eggs
- 1/4 cup all-purpose flour
- 1 tablespoon honey
- 1/2 teaspoon baking powder
- 1/4 teaspoon vanilla extract
- Pinch of salt
- 1 cup fresh blueberries
- 1/4 cup water
- 1 tablespoon lemon juice
- Maple syrup for serving

Instructions:

1. In a blender, combine the cottage cheese, eggs, flour, honey, baking powder, vanilla extract, and salt.

2. Blend until the batter is smooth and well combined.

3. Heat a non-stick skillet over medium heat and lightly grease it with cooking spray or butter.

4. Pour 1/4 cup of the pancake batter onto the skillet to form a pancake.

5. Cook the pancake for 2-3 minutes on each side until it is golden brown and cooked through.

6. Repeat the cooking process with the remaining batter to make more pancakes.

7. In a separate saucepan, combine the blueberries, water, and lemon juice to make the blueberry compote.

8. Cook the compote over medium heat for about 5 minutes or until the blueberries soften and release their juices.

9. Serve the cottage cheese pancakes with the warm blueberry compote and drizzle with maple syrup for added sweetness.

10. Enjoy this delightful and protein-rich pancake breakfast.

Spinach and Mushroom Breakfast Burrito

Ingredients:

- 2 large whole wheat tortillas
- 4 large eggs, beaten
- 1 cup chopped spinach
- 1/2 cup sliced mushrooms
- 1/4 cup diced onions
- 1/4 cup shredded cheddar cheese
- Salt and pepper to taste
- 1 tablespoon olive oil
- Salsa or hot sauce for serving (optional)

Instructions:

1. In a medium-sized skillet, heat the olive oil over medium heat.
2. Add the diced onions and sliced mushrooms to the skillet and sauté until they become tender.

3. Stir in the chopped spinach and cook until wilted.

4. Pour the beaten eggs into the skillet, and scramble them together with the sautéed vegetables until they are cooked through.

5. Season the eggs with salt and pepper to taste.

6. Warm the whole wheat tortillas in a separate pan or in the microwave for a few seconds until they are pliable.

7. Divide the scrambled egg mixture evenly between the two tortillas.

8. Sprinkle shredded cheddar cheese over the eggs.

9. Fold the sides of the tortillas inward, and then roll them up to form a burrito shape.

10. Serve the breakfast burritos as is or with salsa or hot sauce for added flavor and heat.

11. Enjoy this hearty and satisfying breakfast that's perfect for those on the go.

Almond Butter and Banana Sandwich on Whole Grain Bread

Ingredients:

- 4 slices whole grain bread
- 1/2 cup almond butter
- 2 ripe bananas, sliced
- 1 tablespoon honey
- 1 tablespoon chia seeds (optional)

Instructions:

1. Lay out the four slices of whole grain bread on a clean surface.
2. Spread almond butter evenly on two slices of the bread.
3. Layer the sliced bananas on top of the almond butter.
4. Drizzle honey over the bananas for added sweetness.
5. Sprinkle chia seeds on top if desired, for extra nutrition.
6. Place the remaining two slices of bread on top to form sandwiches.

7. Press gently to seal the sandwiches together.

8. Cut the sandwiches diagonally to create four delicious almond butter and banana halves.

9. Serve and enjoy this simple yet satisfying breakfast sandwich.

Chapter 3: Lunch Recipes

In this chapter, we will explore ten tantalizing lunch recipes that are both satisfying and nutritious. From vibrant salads to savory wraps and hearty soups, these lunch options will keep you energized and fueled throughout the day.

Grilled Chicken Salad with Balsamic Vinaigrette

Ingredients:

- 2 boneless, skinless chicken breasts
- 4 cups mixed greens (spinach, arugula, or lettuce of your choice)
- 1 cup cherry tomatoes, halved
- 1/2 cucumber, sliced
- 1/4 red onion, thinly sliced
- 1/4 cup crumbled feta cheese
- 2 tablespoons balsamic vinaigrette dressing
- Salt and pepper to taste

Instructions:

1. Preheat the grill to medium-high heat.

2. Season the chicken breasts with salt and pepper.

3. Grill the chicken for about 5-6 minutes per side or until fully cooked.

4. Let the chicken rest for a few minutes, then slice it into thin strips.

5. In a large bowl, combine the mixed greens, cherry tomatoes, cucumber, and red onion.

6. Top the salad with the sliced grilled chicken and crumbled feta cheese.

7. Drizzle the balsamic vinaigrette dressing over the salad and toss gently to combine.

8. Serve immediately and enjoy the delightful combination of flavors and textures.

Black Bean and Quinoa Salad

Ingredients:

- 1 cup cooked quinoa
- 1 can (15 oz) black beans, drained and rinsed
- 1 cup corn kernels (fresh, frozen, or canned)
- 1 red bell pepper, diced
- 1/4 cup chopped fresh cilantro

- 2 tablespoons lime juice

- 2 tablespoons olive oil

- 1 teaspoon ground cumin

- Salt and pepper to taste

Instructions:

1. In a large mixing bowl, combine the cooked quinoa, black beans, corn, diced red bell pepper, and chopped cilantro.

2. In a separate small bowl, whisk together the lime juice, olive oil, ground cumin, salt, and pepper.

3. Pour the dressing over the quinoa mixture and toss gently to coat everything evenly.

4. Refrigerate the salad for at least 30 minutes before serving to allow the flavors to meld together.

5. This refreshing and protein-packed salad can be enjoyed on its own or served as a side dish with grilled chicken or fish.

Turkey and Avocado Wrap

Ingredients:

- 4 whole wheat or spinach tortillas

- 1/2 pound sliced turkey breast
- 1 avocado, thinly sliced
- 1 cup baby spinach leaves
- 1/4 cup shredded cheddar cheese
- 2 tablespoons ranch dressing

Instructions:

1. Lay the tortillas flat on a clean surface.
2. Evenly divide the sliced turkey, avocado, baby spinach, and shredded cheddar cheese among the tortillas.
3. Drizzle the ranch dressing over the fillings.
4. Roll up the tortillas tightly, tucking in the sides as you go.
5. Slice the wraps in half and serve immediately, or wrap them in parchment paper for an on-the-go lunch option.

Mediterranean Chickpea Salad

Ingredients:

- 2 cups cooked chickpeas (canned or homemade)
- 1 cup diced cucumber

- 1 cup cherry tomatoes, halved
- 1/2 cup pitted Kalamata olives, halved
- 1/4 cup crumbled feta cheese
- 2 tablespoons red wine vinegar
- 2 tablespoons extra-virgin olive oil
- 1 teaspoon dried oregano
- Salt and pepper to taste

Instructions:

1. In a large bowl, combine the cooked chickpeas, diced cucumber, halved cherry tomatoes, and Kalamata olives.
2. In a small bowl, whisk together the red wine vinegar, olive oil, dried oregano, salt, and pepper to make the dressing.
3. Pour the dressing over the chickpea mixture and toss gently to coat everything evenly.
4. Sprinkle the crumbled feta cheese over the top and serve this refreshing Mediterranean salad for a taste of the coast.

Shrimp and Veggie Stir-Fry

Ingredients:

- 1 pound large shrimp, peeled and deveined
- 2 cups broccoli florets
- 1 red bell pepper, thinly sliced
- 1 carrot, julienned
- 1/2 cup snap peas
- 2 tablespoons soy sauce
- 1 tablespoon oyster sauce
- 1 tablespoon sesame oil
- 2 cloves garlic, minced
- 1 teaspoon grated fresh ginger
- 2 green onions, sliced

Instructions:

1. In a small bowl, whisk together the soy sauce, oyster sauce, sesame oil, minced garlic, and grated ginger to make the stir-fry sauce.

2. Heat a large skillet or wok over medium-high heat and add a splash of vegetable oil.

3. Add the shrimp to the skillet and cook for 2-3 minutes until they start to turn pink.

4. Add the broccoli, red bell pepper, carrot, and snap peas to the skillet, stirring constantly.

5. Pour the stir-fry sauce over the shrimp and veggies and continue to cook for another 2-3 minutes until the shrimp are fully cooked and the vegetables are tender-crisp.

6. Sprinkle the sliced green onions over the top and serve this savory and satisfying shrimp and veggie stir-fry with steamed rice or noodles.

Tofu Lettuce Wraps with Peanut Sauce

Ingredients:

- 1 block firm tofu, drained and diced
- 1 tablespoon vegetable oil
- 1/4 cup hoisin sauce
- 2 tablespoons soy sauce
- 1 tablespoon rice vinegar
- 1 tablespoon Sriracha sauce (optional for extra heat)
- 1 tablespoon peanut butter
- 1 teaspoon grated fresh ginger

- 1/4 cup chopped peanuts
- 1 head Boston lettuce, leaves separated

Instructions:

1. Heat the vegetable oil in a large skillet over medium-high heat.
2. Add the diced tofu to the skillet and cook for 4-5 minutes until lightly browned and crispy.
3. In a small bowl, whisk together the hoisin sauce, soy sauce, rice vinegar, Sriracha sauce (if using), peanut butter, and grated ginger to make the peanut sauce.
4. Pour the peanut sauce over the cooked tofu in the skillet and toss to coat evenly.
5. Sprinkle the chopped peanuts over the top.
6. To serve, scoop the tofu mixture into individual Boston lettuce leaves, creating delicious and satisfying lettuce wraps.

Lentil and Vegetable Soup

Ingredients:

- 1 cup dried green lentils, rinsed

- 1 tablespoon olive oil

- 1 onion, diced

- 2 carrots, diced

- 2 celery stalks, diced

- 2 cloves garlic, minced

- 1 teaspoon ground cumin

- 1/2 teaspoon ground turmeric

- 1/4 teaspoon cayenne pepper (optional for a spicy kick)

- 4 cups vegetable broth

- 1 can (14 oz) diced tomatoes

- Salt and pepper to taste

- Fresh parsley, chopped (for garnish)

Instructions:

1. In a large pot, heat the olive oil over medium heat.

2. Add the diced onion, carrots, and celery, and sauté for 5-6 minutes until softened.

3. Stir in the minced garlic, ground cumin, ground turmeric, and cayenne pepper (if using), and cook for another minute until fragrant.

4. Add the rinsed lentils, vegetable broth, and diced tomatoes to the pot.

5. Bring the soup to a boil, then reduce the heat to low and let it simmer for 20-25 minutes until the lentils are tender.

6. Season the soup with salt and pepper to taste.

7. Ladle the hearty lentil and vegetable soup into bowls and garnish with chopped fresh parsley.

Turkey and Sweet Potato Chili

Ingredients:

- 1 tablespoon olive oil
- 1 pound ground turkey
- 1 onion, diced
- 2 cloves garlic, minced
- 1 red bell pepper, diced
- 1 can (15 oz) diced tomatoes
- 1 can (15 oz) black beans, drained and rinsed
- 1 large sweet potato, peeled and diced
- 2 cups chicken broth
- 2 tablespoons chili powder
- 1 teaspoon ground cumin

- Salt and pepper to taste

- Fresh cilantro, chopped (for garnish)

Instructions:

1. In a large pot, heat the olive oil over medium heat.

2. Add the ground turkey to the pot and cook until browned, breaking it apart with a spatula.

3. Stir in the diced onion, minced garlic, and diced red bell pepper, and sauté for 5-6 minutes until the vegetables are softened.

4. Add the diced tomatoes, black beans, diced sweet potato, chicken broth, chili powder, ground cumin, salt, and pepper to the pot.

5. Bring the chili to a boil, then reduce the heat to low and let it simmer for 20-25 minutes until the sweet potatoes are tender and the flavors have melded together.

6. Serve the hearty and comforting turkey and sweet potato chili in bowls and garnish with chopped fresh cilantro.

Falafel Bowl with Hummus and Tabouli

Ingredients:

- 1 cup cooked quinoa or bulgur wheat
- 1 cup falafel balls (store-bought or homemade)
- 1 cup hummus
- 1 cup tabouli salad
- 1/2 cucumber, diced
- 1/4 cup crumbled feta cheese
- Lemon wedges (for serving)

Instructions:

1. In individual serving bowls, arrange the cooked quinoa or bulgur wheat as the base.
2. Top the grain with falafel balls, hummus, and tabouli salad.
3. Add the diced cucumber and sprinkle the crumbled feta cheese over the top.
4. Serve the falafel bowl with a squeeze of fresh lemon juice for a burst of tangy flavor.

Grilled Portobello Mushroom Burger

Ingredients:

- 4 large Portobello mushroom caps
- 2 tablespoons balsamic vinegar
- 2 tablespoons soy sauce
- 2 tablespoons olive oil
- 2 cloves garlic, minced
- 4 whole wheat burger buns
- Lettuce leaves
- Sliced tomatoes
- Sliced red onion
- Avocado slices
- Dijon mustard or your favorite burger sauce

Instructions:

1. Preheat the grill to medium-high heat.
2. In a small bowl, whisk together the balsamic vinegar, soy sauce, olive oil, and minced garlic to make the marinade.
3. Brush the mushroom caps with the marinade, making sure to coat both sides.

4. Grill the mushrooms for 3-4 minutes per side until they are tender and slightly charred.

5. Toast the whole wheat burger buns on the grill for a minute or until they are warm and lightly toasted.

6. Assemble the grilled Portobello mushroom burgers by placing a mushroom cap on each bun.

7. Top with lettuce leaves, sliced tomatoes, sliced red onion, and avocado slices.

8. Spread a dollop of Dijon mustard or your favorite burger sauce on the top bun.

9. Serve these mouthwatering grilled Portobello mushroom burgers alongside a fresh side salad or sweet potato fries.

Chapter 4: Dinner Recipes

In this chapter, we will explore an enticing array of dinner recipes that are not only delicious but also packed with nutrients to fuel your body. These dinners will be the perfect way to end your day with a satisfying and wholesome meal.

Baked Salmon with Asparagus and Lemon

Ingredients:

- 4 salmon fillets
- 1 bunch of fresh asparagus
- 2 lemons (1 sliced, 1 juiced)
- 2 tablespoons of olive oil
- 2 cloves of garlic, minced
- 1 teaspoon of dried thyme
- Salt and pepper to taste

Instructions:

1. Preheat your oven to 375°F (190°C).

2. Place the salmon fillets on a baking sheet lined with parchment paper.

3. Arrange the asparagus spears around the salmon on the same baking sheet.

4. Drizzle olive oil over the salmon and asparagus, making sure they are evenly coated.

5. Sprinkle minced garlic, dried thyme, salt, and pepper over the salmon and asparagus.

6. Place lemon slices on top of each salmon fillet.

7. Squeeze fresh lemon juice over the entire dish.

8. Bake in the preheated oven for 15-20 minutes or until the salmon is cooked through and flakes easily with a fork.

9. Serve the Baked Salmon with Asparagus and Lemon with a side of quinoa or brown rice for a complete and wholesome meal.

Lemon Herb Grilled Chicken with Roasted Vegetables

Ingredients:

- 4 boneless, skinless chicken breasts

- 2 tablespoons of olive oil

- 1 lemon (zested and juiced)

- 2 cloves of garlic, minced

- 1 teaspoon of dried oregano

- 1 teaspoon of dried thyme

- Salt and pepper to taste

- Assorted vegetables (such as bell peppers, zucchini, and red onions), sliced

Instructions:

1. In a bowl, mix together olive oil, lemon zest, lemon juice, minced garlic, dried oregano, dried thyme, salt, and pepper to create the marinade.

2. Place the chicken breasts in the marinade and let them marinate for at least 30 minutes.

3. Preheat your grill to medium-high heat.

4. Grill the marinated chicken breasts for about 6-8 minutes per side or until they reach an internal temperature of 165°F (74°C).

5. While the chicken is grilling, toss the sliced vegetables in a separate bowl with a drizzle of olive oil, salt, and pepper.

6. Roast the seasoned vegetables in the oven at 400°F (200°C) for 15-20 minutes or until they are tender and slightly caramelized.

7. Serve the Lemon Herb Grilled Chicken with Roasted Vegetables for a delightful and healthy dinner option.

Spaghetti Squash with Marinara and Turkey Meatballs

Ingredients:

- 1 medium-sized spaghetti squash
- 1 pound of ground turkey
- 1/2 cup of breadcrumbs
- 1/4 cup of grated Parmesan cheese
- 1 egg, lightly beaten
- 2 cups of marinara sauce
- 2 tablespoons of olive oil
- 2 cloves of garlic, minced
- 1 teaspoon of dried basil
- Salt and pepper to taste

Instructions:

1. Preheat your oven to 400°F (200°C).

2. Cut the spaghetti squash in half lengthwise and scoop out the seeds.

3. Place the squash halves, cut side down, on a baking sheet lined with parchment paper.

4. Bake the spaghetti squash in the preheated oven for 35-40 minutes or until it becomes tender and can be easily shredded with a fork.

5. While the squash is baking, prepare the turkey meatballs by combining ground turkey, breadcrumbs, grated Parmesan cheese, lightly beaten egg, dried basil, salt, and pepper in a bowl. Mix well and form small meatballs.

6. Heat olive oil in a skillet over medium heat. Add minced garlic and cook until fragrant.

7. Add the turkey meatballs to the skillet and cook until they are browned on all sides and cooked through.

8. Pour the marinara sauce over the meatballs and let it simmer for a few minutes.

9. Once the spaghetti squash is done, use a fork to shred the flesh into spaghetti-like strands.

10. Serve the Spaghetti Squash with Marinara and Turkey Meatballs for a wholesome and satisfying dinner.

Zucchini Noodles with Pesto and Cherry Tomatoes

Ingredients:

- 4 medium-sized zucchinis, spiralized into noodles
- 1 cup of fresh basil leaves
- 1/2 cup of pine nuts
- 1/2 cup of grated Parmesan cheese
- 2 cloves of garlic
- 1/2 cup of extra-virgin olive oil
- 1 cup of cherry tomatoes, halved
- Salt and pepper to taste

Instructions:

1. In a food processor, combine fresh basil, pine nuts, grated Parmesan cheese, garlic, salt, and pepper.

2. Pulse the ingredients while slowly adding the olive oil until the pesto reaches your desired consistency.

3. In a large skillet, sauté the zucchini noodles over medium heat until they are tender but not mushy.

4. Toss the zucchini noodles with the prepared pesto until they are well coated.

5. Add the halved cherry tomatoes to the zucchini noodles and gently toss them together.

6. Serve the Zucchini Noodles with Pesto and Cherry Tomatoes for a flavorful and low-carb dinner option.

Beef Stir-Fry with Broccoli and Snow Peas

Ingredients:

- 1 pound of beef sirloin, thinly sliced
- 2 tablespoons of soy sauce
- 2 tablespoons of oyster sauce
- 1 tablespoon of cornstarch
- 2 tablespoons of vegetable oil
- 2 cloves of garlic, minced

- 1-inch piece of ginger, grated
- 2 cups of broccoli florets
- 1 cup of snow peas
- 1 red bell pepper, thinly sliced
- 1 tablespoon of sesame oil
- Sesame seeds for garnish (optional)

Instructions:

1. In a bowl, mix together soy sauce, oyster sauce, and cornstarch to create the marinade.
2. Add the thinly sliced beef to the marinade and let it marinate for at least 15 minutes.
3. In a large skillet or wok, heat vegetable oil over medium-high heat.
4. Stir-fry the marinated beef until it is browned and cooked to your desired level of doneness. Remove the beef from the skillet and set it aside.
5. In the same skillet, add minced garlic and grated ginger, and stir-fry for about 30 seconds until fragrant.

6. Add broccoli florets, snow peas, and sliced red bell
    pepper to the skillet, and stir-fry until they are
    tender-crisp.

7. Return the cooked beef to the skillet and toss it with
    the vegetables.

8. Drizzle sesame oil over the stir-fry and toss it to
    coat evenly.

9. Garnish with sesame seeds if desired, and serve the
    Beef Stir-Fry with Broccoli and Snow Peas over a
    bed of brown rice or quinoa for a hearty and
    flavorful dinner.

Cauliflower Rice Stir-Fry with Tofu and Cashews

Ingredients:

- 1 medium-sized cauliflower head, riced
- 1 block of firm tofu, cubed
- 1 cup of broccoli florets
- 1 cup of sliced carrots
- 1/2 cup of chopped green onions
- 1/2 cup of cashews

- 3 tablespoons of soy sauce

- 2 tablespoons of hoisin sauce

- 1 tablespoon of sesame oil

- 2 cloves of garlic, minced

- 1-inch piece of ginger, grated

- Salt and pepper to taste

Instructions:

1. In a large skillet or wok, heat sesame oil over medium heat.

2. Add minced garlic and grated ginger, and stir-fry for about 30 seconds until fragrant.

3. Add cubed tofu to the skillet and stir-fry until it becomes lightly browned and crispy on all sides.

4. Push the tofu to one side of the skillet and add broccoli florets and sliced carrots to the other side. Stir-fry the vegetables until they are tender-crisp.

5. Mix the tofu and vegetables together in the skillet, and then add the cauliflower rice to the mixture.

6. Pour soy sauce and hoisin sauce over the cauliflower rice and tofu, and stir-fry everything until the flavors are well combined.

7. Toss in chopped green onions and cashews, and stir-fry for an additional minute.

8. Season the Cauliflower Rice Stir-Fry with Tofu and Cashews with salt and pepper to taste.

9. Serve this delicious and nutritious stir-fry for a satisfying and healthy dinner option.

Stuffed Bell Peppers with Quinoa and Black Beans

Ingredients:

- 4 bell peppers (any color), halved and seeds removed
- 1 cup of cooked quinoa
- 1 can (15 ounces) of black beans, drained and rinsed
- 1 cup of diced tomatoes
- 1 cup of corn kernels (fresh, frozen, or canned)
- 1/2 cup of diced red onion
- 1 teaspoon of ground cumin
- 1 teaspoon of chili powder
- Salt and pepper to taste
- 1/2 cup of shredded cheddar cheese (optional)

Instructions:

1. Preheat your oven to 375°F (190°C).
2. In a large bowl, mix together cooked quinoa, black beans, diced tomatoes, corn kernels, diced red onion, ground cumin, chili powder, salt, and pepper.
3. Stuff each bell pepper half with the quinoa and black bean mixture.
4. Place the stuffed bell peppers in a baking dish and cover the dish with aluminum foil.
5. Bake in the preheated oven for 25-30 minutes or until the bell peppers are tender.
6. If desired, sprinkle shredded cheddar cheese on top of each stuffed bell pepper during the last 5 minutes of baking for a cheesy twist.
7. Serve the Stuffed Bell Peppers with Quinoa and Black Beans for a colorful and nutritious dinner.

Baked Cod with Steamed Green Beans

Ingredients:

- 4 cod fillets

- 2 tablespoons of olive oil

- 1 tablespoon of lemon juice

- 1 teaspoon of dried oregano

- 1 teaspoon of dried thyme

- Salt and pepper to taste

- 1 pound of fresh green beans, trimmed

Instructions:

1. Preheat your oven to 400°F (200°C).

2. Place the cod fillets on a baking sheet lined with parchment paper.

3. Drizzle olive oil and lemon juice over the cod fillets, ensuring they are evenly coated.

4. Sprinkle dried oregano, dried thyme, salt, and pepper over the cod fillets.

5. Bake the cod in the preheated oven for 12-15 minutes or until it is opaque and flakes easily with a fork.

6. While the cod is baking, steam the trimmed green beans until they are tender-crisp.

7. Serve the Baked Cod with Steamed Green Beans for a light and wholesome dinner option.

Eggplant Parmesan with Mixed Greens Salad

Ingredients:

- 2 medium-sized eggplants, sliced
- 1 cup of all-purpose flour
- 2 eggs, lightly beaten
- 2 cups of breadcrumbs
- 1 cup of grated Parmesan cheese
- 2 cups of marinara sauce
- 2 cups of shredded mozzarella cheese
- 1 tablespoon of dried basil
- 1 tablespoon of dried oregano
- Salt and pepper to taste
- Mixed greens salad (arugula, spinach, and kale) for serving

Instructions:

1. Preheat your oven to 375°F (190°C).
2. Dredge the eggplant slices in all-purpose flour, then dip them in the beaten eggs, and finally coat them in breadcrumbs mixed with grated Parmesan cheese, dried basil, dried oregano, salt, and pepper.

3. Place the coated eggplant slices on a baking sheet lined with parchment paper and bake in the preheated oven for 20-25 minutes or until they are golden and crispy.
4. In a baking dish, spread a layer of marinara sauce on the bottom.
5. Arrange the baked eggplant slices on top of the sauce.
6. Sprinkle shredded mozzarella cheese over the eggplant slices, and then add another layer of marinara sauce.
7. Repeat the layers with the remaining eggplant, cheese, and sauce until all the ingredients are used.
8. Finish with a generous layer of mozzarella cheese on top.
9. Bake the Eggplant Parmesan in the oven for 25-30 minutes or until the cheese is bubbly and golden.
10. Serve the Eggplant Parmesan with a side of mixed greens salad for a delightful and satisfying dinner.

Thai Green Curry with Tofu and Cauliflower Rice

Ingredients:

- 1 block of firm tofu, cubed
- 1 tablespoon of vegetable oil
- 2 tablespoons of green curry paste
- 1 can (14 ounces) of coconut milk
- 1 cup of vegetable broth
- 2 cups of assorted vegetables (such as bell peppers, carrots, and broccoli), sliced
- 1 cup of cauliflower rice
- 1 tablespoon of soy sauce
- 1 tablespoon of brown sugar
- Fresh cilantro for garnish (optional)

Instructions:

1. In a large skillet or wok, heat vegetable oil over medium heat.
2. Add cubed tofu to the skillet and stir-fry until it becomes lightly browned and crispy on all sides.
3. Add green curry paste to the skillet and stir-fry for about 1 minute until fragrant.

4. Pour in coconut milk and vegetable broth, and stir to combine the ingredients.

5. Add the sliced assorted vegetables to the curry mixture and let them simmer until they are tender.

6. Meanwhile, in a separate skillet, cook the cauliflower rice until it becomes tender but not mushy.

7. Add soy sauce and brown sugar to the curry mixture and adjust the seasoning to your taste.

8. Serve the Thai Green Curry with Tofu and Cauliflower Rice, garnished with fresh cilantro if desired, for a flavorful and exotic dinner option.

Chapter 5: Snacks and Appetizers

In this chapter, we explore ten delicious and nutritious snacks and appetizers that will satisfy your cravings without derailing your 30-day macro diet meal plan.

Veggie Sticks with Hummus

Ingredients:

- Carrot sticks
- Celery sticks
- Cucumber sticks
- Cherry tomatoes
- Red bell pepper strips
- Homemade hummus (recipe below)

Instructions:

1. Wash and cut the veggies into sticks or strips.
2. Arrange the colorful veggie sticks on a platter.
3. Serve with a bowl of homemade hummus.

Homemade Hummus:

Ingredients:

- 1 can of chickpeas, drained and rinsed
- 2 cloves of garlic
- 3 tablespoons of tahini
- 3 tablespoons of lemon juice
- 2 tablespoons of olive oil
- 1/2 teaspoon of ground cumin
- Salt and pepper to taste
- Water (as needed for desired consistency)

Instructions:

1. In a food processor, blend the chickpeas, garlic, tahini, lemon juice, and olive oil until smooth.
2. Add ground cumin, salt, and pepper. Blend again to combine.
3. If the hummus is too thick, add water gradually until you achieve the desired creamy consistency.

Greek Yogurt with Cucumber and Dill Dip

Ingredients:

- 1 cup of Greek yogurt
- 1/2 cucumber, finely diced
- 1 tablespoon of fresh dill, chopped
- 1 clove of garlic, minced
- Salt and pepper to taste

Instructions:

1. In a mixing bowl, combine Greek yogurt, diced cucumber, fresh dill, minced garlic, salt, and pepper.
2. Stir well until all ingredients are evenly distributed.
3. Refrigerate for at least 30 minutes before serving to allow flavors to meld.

Sliced Apple with Almond Butter

Ingredients:

- Apples (your choice of variety)
- Almond butter

Instructions:

1. Wash and slice the apples into thin wedges.

2. Arrange the apple slices on a plate.

3. Serve with a side of almond butter for dipping.

Rice Cakes with Avocado and Sprouts

Ingredients:

- Rice cakes

- Ripe avocado

- Fresh sprouts (alfalfa, broccoli, or any of your preference)

- Lemon juice

- Salt and pepper to taste

Instructions:

1. Cut the avocado in half, remove the pit, and scoop out the flesh into a bowl.

2. Mash the avocado with a fork and season with lemon juice, salt, and pepper to taste.

3. Spread the avocado mixture on rice cakes.

4. Top with fresh sprouts for added crunch and
    nutrition.

Edamame with Sea Salt

Ingredients:

- Edamame (fresh or frozen)
- Sea salt

Instructions:

1. Boil the edamame pods in salted water until tender.
2. Drain and sprinkle with sea salt.
3. Serve warm as a delicious and protein-packed
    snack.

Guacamole and Salsa with Baked Tortilla Chips

Ingredients:

Guacamole:

- 2 ripe avocados
- 1/4 cup of diced red onion
- 1 small tomato, diced

- 1 jalapeno pepper, seeded and minced (optional)
- 2 tablespoons of fresh cilantro, chopped
- 1 tablespoon of lime juice
- Salt and pepper to taste

Salsa:

- 2 cups of diced tomatoes
- 1/4 cup of diced red onion
- 1 jalapeno pepper, seeded and minced
- 2 tablespoons of fresh cilantro, chopped
- 1 tablespoon of lime juice
- Salt and pepper to taste

Baked Tortilla Chips:

- Whole-grain tortillas
- Olive oil
- Salt

Instructions:

Guacamole:

1. In a mixing bowl, mash the ripe avocados with a fork.

2. Add diced red onion, tomato, jalapeno (if using), and chopped cilantro.

3. Squeeze in lime juice, season with salt and pepper, and mix well.

Salsa:

1. Combine diced tomatoes, red onion, minced jalapeno, and chopped cilantro in a bowl.

2. Add lime juice, salt, and pepper, and toss until well combined.

Baked Tortilla Chips:

1. Preheat your oven to 350°F (175°C).

2. Brush whole-grain tortillas with olive oil on both sides.

3. Sprinkle with salt and cut into triangle wedges.

4. Arrange the tortilla wedges on a baking sheet and bake for about 10-12 minutes or until crispy.

Cottage Cheese and Pineapple Chunks

Ingredients:

- Cottage cheese
- Fresh pineapple, cut into chunks

Instructions:

1. Place a scoop of cottage cheese in a serving bowl.
2. Add fresh pineapple chunks on top.
3. Enjoy this creamy and fruity combination as a satisfying snack.

Mixed Nuts and Seeds Trail Mix

Ingredients:

- Almonds
- Cashews
- Walnuts
- Pumpkin seeds
- Sunflower seeds
- Dried cranberries (or any other dried fruit of your choice)

- Dark chocolate chips (optional)

Instructions:

1. In a bowl, combine almonds, cashews, walnuts, pumpkin seeds, sunflower seeds, and dried cranberries.
2. Optionally, add dark chocolate chips for a touch of sweetness.
3. Mix well and store in an airtight container for a convenient on-the-go snack.

Carrot and Zucchini Fritters

Ingredients:

- 2 cups of shredded carrots
- 1 cup of shredded zucchini
- 1/4 cup of whole wheat flour
- 2 eggs, lightly beaten
- 1/4 cup of grated Parmesan cheese
- 2 tablespoons of chopped fresh parsley
- 1 clove of garlic, minced
- Salt and pepper to taste
- Olive oil for frying

Instructions:

1. In a large bowl, combine shredded carrots, zucchini, whole wheat flour, beaten eggs, grated Parmesan cheese, chopped parsley, minced garlic, salt, and pepper.
2. Mix until all ingredients are well incorporated.
3. Heat olive oil in a skillet over medium heat.
4. Drop spoonfuls of the mixture onto the hot skillet and flatten with a spatula.
5. Cook until fritters are golden brown on both sides.
6. Serve warm and enjoy this delicious and veggie-packed snack.

Stuffed Mini Bell Peppers with Goat Cheese

Ingredients:

- Mini bell peppers (various colors)
- Goat cheese
- Fresh basil leaves
- Balsamic glaze (optional)

Instructions:

1. Cut the tops off the mini bell peppers and remove the seeds.

2. Fill each pepper with goat cheese and top with a fresh basil leaf.

3. Arrange the stuffed mini bell peppers on a serving plate.

4. Optionally, drizzle with balsamic glaze for an extra burst of flavor.

Chapter 6: Desserts

Mixed Berry Parfait with Greek Yogurt

Ingredients:

- 1 cup mixed berries (strawberries, blueberries, raspberries)
- 1 cup Greek yogurt
- 1 tablespoon honey
- 1/4 cup granola

Instructions:

1. Wash the mixed berries thoroughly and pat them dry.
2. In a bowl, mix Greek yogurt with honey until well combined.
3. In a glass or parfait dish, layer the yogurt mixture, mixed berries, and granola.
4. Repeat the layers until the glass is filled.
5. Top with a few more berries and a drizzle of honey.

6. Serve immediately or refrigerate for a few hours to let the flavors meld.

Chocolate Protein Balls with Almond Butter

Ingredients:

- 1 cup rolled oats
- 1/2 cup almond butter
- 1/4 cup honey
- 1/4 cup chocolate protein powder
- 1/4 cup dark chocolate chips
- 1 teaspoon vanilla extract
- Pinch of salt

Instructions:

1. In a large mixing bowl, combine rolled oats, almond butter, honey, chocolate protein powder, dark chocolate chips, vanilla extract, and a pinch of salt.
2. Mix until the ingredients form a sticky dough.
3. Take small portions of the dough and roll them into bite-sized balls using your hands.

4. Place the balls on a baking sheet lined with parchment paper.

5. Refrigerate the balls for at least 30 minutes to firm up before serving.

Frozen Banana Popsicles with Dark Chocolate Drizzle

Ingredients:

- 2 ripe bananas
- 1/2 cup dark chocolate chips
- 2 tablespoons coconut oil
- Assorted toppings (chopped nuts, shredded coconut, sprinkles)

Instructions:

1. Peel the bananas and cut them in half.

2. Insert popsicle sticks into the cut ends of the bananas.

3. Place the bananas on a parchment-lined baking sheet and freeze for at least 2 hours.

4. In a microwave-safe bowl, melt the dark chocolate chips and coconut oil in short intervals, stirring until smooth.

5. Dip each frozen banana into the melted chocolate, then quickly sprinkle with toppings of your choice.

6. Place the coated bananas back on the baking sheet and freeze for another hour or until the chocolate hardens.

Baked Apples with Cinnamon and Greek Yogurt

Ingredients:

- 4 medium-sized apples (Honeycrisp or Granny Smith)
- 2 tablespoons melted butter
- 2 tablespoons honey
- 1 teaspoon ground cinnamon
- 1 cup Greek yogurt

Instructions:

1. Preheat the oven to 375°F (190°C).

2. Core the apples and make a shallow cut around the middle to prevent bursting.

3. In a small bowl, mix melted butter, honey, and ground cinnamon.

4. Brush the mixture over the apples, making sure to coat them evenly.

5. Place the apples in a baking dish and bake for about 30 minutes or until they are tender.

6. Serve the baked apples with a dollop of Greek yogurt on top.

Chia Seed Chocolate Pudding

Ingredients:

- 1/4 cup chia seeds
- 1 cup almond milk
- 2 tablespoons unsweetened cocoa powder
- 2 tablespoons maple syrup
- 1 teaspoon vanilla extract

Instructions:

1. In a bowl, mix chia seeds, almond milk, cocoa powder, maple syrup, and vanilla extract.

2. Stir the mixture well until the chia seeds are evenly distributed.

3. Cover the bowl and refrigerate for at least 4 hours or overnight to allow the chia seeds to absorb the liquid and thicken into a pudding-like consistency.

4. Serve chilled and top with fresh berries if desired.

Coconut and Date Energy Bites

Ingredients:

- 1 cup shredded coconut (unsweetened)
- 1 cup pitted dates
- 1/2 cup almonds
- 1/4 cup almond butter
- 1 tablespoon honey
- 1 teaspoon vanilla extract

Instructions:

1. In a food processor, combine shredded coconut, pitted dates, almonds, almond butter, honey, and vanilla extract.

2. Pulse the mixture until it forms a sticky and crumbly dough.

3. Take small portions of the dough and roll them into bite-sized balls using your hands.

4. Place the energy bites on a plate and refrigerate for at least 30 minutes to firm up before serving.

Peanut Butter and Banana Frozen Bites

Ingredients:

- 2 ripe bananas
- 1/4 cup peanut butter
- 1/4 cup dark chocolate chips
- 1 teaspoon coconut oil
- Crushed peanuts (optional)

Instructions:

1. Peel the bananas and cut them into thick slices.

2. Spread peanut butter on half of the banana slices and then top with the remaining slices to make a sandwich.

3. Place the banana sandwiches on a baking sheet
   lined with parchment paper and freeze for at least 2
   hours.
4. In a microwave-safe bowl, melt the dark chocolate
   chips and coconut oil in short intervals, stirring until
   smooth.
5. Dip each frozen banana sandwich into the melted
   chocolate, then quickly sprinkle with crushed
   peanuts if desired.
6. Place the coated banana bites back on the baking
   sheet and freeze for another hour or until the
   chocolate hardens.

Berry Chia Seed Jam on Whole Grain Toast

Ingredients:

- 2 cups mixed berries (strawberries, blueberries, raspberries)
- 2 tablespoons chia seeds
- 2 tablespoons honey
- 1 tablespoon lemon juice

- Whole grain bread slices

Instructions:

1. In a saucepan, combine mixed berries, chia seeds, honey, and lemon juice.
2. Cook over medium heat, stirring occasionally until the berries break down and the mixture thickens into jam-like consistency (about 10 minutes).
3. Remove from heat and let the jam cool down.
4. Spread the berry chia seed jam over whole grain toast and enjoy as a healthy dessert or snack.

Almond Flour Chocolate Chip Cookies

Ingredients:

- 1 cup almond flour
- 1/4 cup coconut oil (melted)
- 1/4 cup maple syrup
- 1 teaspoon vanilla extract
- 1/2 teaspoon baking soda
- Pinch of salt

- 1/2 cup dark chocolate chips

Instructions:

1. Preheat the oven to 350°F (175°C) and line a baking sheet with parchment paper.
2. In a bowl, mix almond flour, melted coconut oil, maple syrup, vanilla extract, baking soda, and a pinch of salt until a smooth batter forms.
3. Stir in dark chocolate chips until evenly distributed.
4. Scoop tablespoons of the cookie dough onto the prepared baking sheet, leaving space between each cookie.
5. Flatten the dough slightly with your fingers or a fork.
6. Bake the cookies for about 10-12 minutes or until the edges turn golden brown.
7. Let the cookies cool on the baking sheet for a few minutes before transferring them to a wire rack to cool completely.

Greek Yogurt and Mixed Berries Sorbet

Ingredients:

- 2 cups mixed berries (strawberries, blueberries, raspberries)
- 1 cup Greek yogurt
- 2 tablespoons honey
- 1 tablespoon lemon juice

Instructions:

1. In a blender or food processor, combine mixed berries, Greek yogurt, honey, and lemon juice.
2. Blend until the mixture is smooth and well combined.
3. Pour the mixture into a shallow dish or ice cream maker and freeze for about 2 hours, stirring every 30 minutes to prevent ice crystals from forming.
4. Once the sorbet reaches the desired consistency, serve in individual bowls or glasses and garnish with fresh berries.

Chapter 7: Smoothies

In this chapter, we will explore ten delectable smoothie recipes that are not only delicious but also packed with health benefits. From the classic Green Spinach and Banana Smoothie to the exotic Tropical Mango and Pineapple Smoothie, these recipes cater to a variety of tastes and preferences.

Green Spinach and Banana Smoothie

Ingredients:

- 1 ripe banana
- 1 cup fresh spinach leaves
- 1/2 cup almond milk
- 1/2 cup Greek yogurt
- 1 tablespoon honey (optional)
- 1/2 teaspoon vanilla extract
- Ice cubes (optional)

Instructions:

1. Peel the banana and place it in the blender.

2. Add the fresh spinach leaves to the blender.

3. Pour in the almond milk and Greek yogurt.

4. Optionally, add a tablespoon of honey for a touch of sweetness.

5. Include the vanilla extract to enhance the flavor.

6. If you prefer a colder smoothie, add a few ice cubes.

7. Blend all the ingredients until smooth and creamy.

8. Pour the Green Spinach and Banana Smoothie into a glass and enjoy its wholesome goodness!

Berry Blast Smoothie with Greek Yogurt

Ingredients:

- 1 cup mixed berries (strawberries, blueberries, raspberries)
- 1/2 cup Greek yogurt
- 1/2 cup orange juice
- 1 tablespoon chia seeds
- 1 tablespoon honey (optional)
- Ice cubes (optional)

Instructions:

1. Wash the mixed berries thoroughly and place them in the blender.
2. Add the Greek yogurt to the berries.
3. Pour in the orange juice for a tangy twist.
4. Include chia seeds to add a boost of fiber and omega-3s.
5. Optionally, add a tablespoon of honey if you desire more sweetness.
6. For a colder texture, toss in a few ice cubes.
7. Blend all the ingredients until the smoothie reaches a delightful consistency.
8. Pour the Berry Blast Smoothie into a glass, and enjoy the burst of fruity flavors!

Tropical Mango and Pineapple Smoothie

Ingredients:

- 1 ripe mango, peeled and diced
- 1 cup fresh pineapple chunks
- 1/2 cup coconut milk

- 1/2 cup orange juice

- 1 tablespoon lime juice

- 1 tablespoon shredded coconut (optional)

- Ice cubes (optional)

Instructions:

1. Prepare the ripe mango by peeling and dicing it.

2. Cut fresh pineapple into chunks and add them to the blender.

3. Pour in the creamy coconut milk for a tropical touch.

4. Include the tangy orange juice and lime juice.

5. Optionally, add shredded coconut to enhance the tropical flavor.

6. For a chilled delight, toss in a few ice cubes.

7. Blend all the ingredients until the smoothie achieves a velvety texture.

8. Pour the Tropical Mango and Pineapple Smoothie into a glass, and indulge in its sunny taste!

Chocolate Banana Protein Smoothie

Ingredients:

- 1 ripe banana
- 2 tablespoons cocoa powder
- 1/2 cup plain Greek yogurt
- 1 cup milk (regular or almond milk)
- 1 tablespoon almond butter
- 1 tablespoon honey (optional)
- Ice cubes (optional)

Instructions:

1. Peel the ripe banana and place it in the blender.
2. Add cocoa powder to create the chocolaty goodness.
3. Pour in the plain Greek yogurt for a protein punch.
4. Choose either regular or almond milk as your liquid base.
5. Include almond butter to enrich the flavor and add healthy fats.
6. Optionally, add a tablespoon of honey if you crave a sweeter taste.
7. For a frosty treat, add a few ice cubes.

8. Blend all the ingredients until the smoothie becomes rich and creamy.

9. Pour the Chocolate Banana Protein Smoothie into a glass, and savor the delightful blend of chocolate and banana!

Blueberry Almond Milk Smoothie

Ingredients:

- 1 cup fresh or frozen blueberries
- 1/2 cup almond milk
- 1/2 cup plain Greek yogurt
- 1 tablespoon almond butter
- 1 tablespoon honey (optional)
- 1/2 teaspoon vanilla extract
- Ice cubes (optional)

Instructions:

1. Wash the blueberries and place them in the blender.

2. Pour in the almond milk for a creamy texture.

3. Add plain Greek yogurt to enhance the smoothie's protein content.

4. Include almond butter to add a nutty twist and healthy fats.

5. Optionally, add a tablespoon of honey for a touch of sweetness.

6. Include vanilla extract to elevate the flavor profile.

7. For an icy refreshment, toss in a few ice cubes.

8. Blend all the ingredients until the smoothie reaches a luscious consistency.

9. Pour the Blueberry Almond Milk Smoothie into a glass, and enjoy the burst of blueberry goodness!

Kale and Kiwi Smoothie

Ingredients:

- 1 cup chopped kale leaves (stems removed)
- 1 ripe kiwi, peeled and sliced
- 1/2 cup pineapple chunks
- 1/2 cup cucumber slices
- 1/2 cup coconut water
- 1 tablespoon lime juice
- 1 tablespoon honey (optional)
- Ice cubes (optional)

Instructions:

1. Wash and chop the kale leaves, removing the stems.
2. Peel and slice the ripe kiwi, and place it in the blender.
3. Add the pineapple chunks and cucumber slices to the blender.
4. Pour in the hydrating coconut water for a tropical touch.
5. Include lime juice to add a zesty kick.
6. Optionally, add a tablespoon of honey if you desire extra sweetness.
7. For a refreshing chill, toss in a few ice cubes.
8. Blend all the ingredients until the smoothie achieves a velvety texture.
9. Pour the Kale and Kiwi Smoothie into a glass, and relish its invigorating flavors!

Peanut Butter and Banana Protein Shake

Ingredients:

- 1 ripe banana

- 2 tablespoons peanut butter

- 1/2 cup milk (regular or almond milk)

- 1/2 cup plain Greek yogurt

- 1 tablespoon honey (optional)

- 1/2 teaspoon cinnamon

- Ice cubes (optional)

Instructions:

1. Peel the ripe banana and place it in the blender.

2. Add peanut butter to impart its rich flavor and protein content.

3. Pour in your choice of milk for the desired consistency.

4. Add plain Greek yogurt for a protein boost.

5. Optionally, add a tablespoon of honey for a sweeter taste.

6. Include a dash of cinnamon to enhance the flavor profile.

7. For a cool treat, toss in a few ice cubes.

8. Blend all the ingredients until the smoothie becomes smooth and creamy.

9. Pour the Peanut Butter and Banana Protein Shake
    into a glass, and savor the delightful blend of peanut
    butter and banana!

Avocado and Spinach Smoothie

Ingredients:

- 1 ripe avocado, peeled and pitted
- 1 cup fresh spinach leaves
- 1/2 cup almond milk
- 1/2 cup Greek yogurt
- 1 tablespoon honey (optional)
- 1 tablespoon lime juice
- Ice cubes (optional)

Instructions:

1. Prepare the ripe avocado by peeling and removing
   the pit.
2. Add the fresh spinach leaves to the blender.
3. Pour in the almond milk and Greek yogurt for a
   creamy texture.
4. Optionally, add a tablespoon of honey if you prefer
   a sweeter taste.

5. Include lime juice to add a zesty kick.

6. For a cool and refreshing blend, toss in a few ice cubes.

7. Blend all the ingredients until the smoothie reaches a delightful consistency.

8. Pour the Avocado and Spinach Smoothie into a glass, and relish its creamy and nutritious goodness!

Raspberry and Coconut Milk Smoothie

Ingredients:

- 1 cup fresh raspberries
- 1/2 cup coconut milk
- 1/2 cup Greek yogurt
- 1 tablespoon chia seeds
- 1 tablespoon honey (optional)
- 1/2 teaspoon vanilla extract
- Ice cubes (optional)

Instructions:

1. Wash the fresh raspberries and place them in the blender.
2. Pour in the luscious coconut milk for a tropical twist.
3. Add Greek yogurt to enhance the smoothie's protein content.
4. Include chia seeds to add a boost of fiber and omega-3s.
5. Optionally, add a tablespoon of honey for extra sweetness.
6. Include vanilla extract to elevate the flavor profile.
7. For a frosty delight, toss in a few ice cubes.
8. Blend all the ingredients until the smoothie achieves a velvety texture.
9. Pour the Raspberry and Coconut Milk Smoothie into a glass, and relish the fusion of raspberry and coconut flavors!

Orange Carrot and Ginger Smoothie

Ingredients:

- 1 cup fresh orange juice
- 1/2 cup chopped carrots

- 1/2 cup Greek yogurt
- 1 tablespoon fresh ginger, grated
- 1 tablespoon honey (optional)
- 1/2 teaspoon turmeric powder (optional)
- Ice cubes (optional)

Instructions:

1. Extract fresh orange juice and place it in the blender.
2. Chop the carrots into smaller pieces and add them to the blender.
3. Pour in Greek yogurt to enhance the smoothie's creaminess.
4. Grate fresh ginger and include it for a zesty kick.
5. Optionally, add a tablespoon of honey if you desire extra sweetness.
6. Optionally, include turmeric powder for its health benefits and color.
7. For a refreshing chill, toss in a few ice cubes.
8. Blend all the ingredients until the smoothie reaches a delightful consistency.

9. Pour the Orange Carrot and Ginger Smoothie into a glass, and enjoy its refreshing citrus taste with a touch of warmth from the ginger!

CONCLUSION

As we conclude this chapter, I want to emphasize the importance of listening to your body and understanding its needs. Your nutritional requirements may change over time, depending on your activity levels, age, and overall health. Be open to adjustments in your meal plan to ensure it remains personalized and effective.

One valuable takeaway from this experience is the significance of meal preparation and planning. By dedicating time to plan your meals and snacks ahead of time, you can avoid impulsive food choices and stay on course with your dietary goals.

Furthermore, always remember that the Macro Diet is not about restricting yourself from indulging in occasional treats. It's all about finding balance and enjoying the journey without guilt. Allow yourself to savor that occasional dessert or favorite comfort food, but always ensure that it fits within your overall nutrition plan.

To continue thriving on this path, staying physically active is equally vital. Regular exercise complements a balanced diet and contributes to your overall well-being. Whether it's going for a brisk walk, engaging in strength training, or practicing yoga, finding an activity you love will make the journey even more enjoyable.

Another crucial aspect of a healthy lifestyle is getting enough restorative sleep. Quality sleep plays a significant role in your body's recovery and rejuvenation process. Aim for seven to nine hours of sleep each night to wake up refreshed and ready to tackle the day with renewed energy.

Thank you for joining us on this transformative journey. May you continue to embrace a life filled with good health, happiness, and abundance.